DASH DIET COOKBOOK AND GUIDE

50 DASH-FRIENDLY RECIPES FOR A BALANCED AND HEALTHY DIET

Table of Contents

Introduction

The Dash diet (Dietary Approaches to Stop Hypertension) speaks clearly with its name already. It is a dietary model created with the aim of improving the health of those who follow it, in particular to combat high blood pressure. It was developed by Harvard University and immediately met with great success in the United States, from there it quickly spread to the rest of the world and became very fashionable all over the world too!

The term "diet" is to a certain extent misleading, since those who want to lower their blood pressure and take advantage of the positive effect of a dietary change must above all try to change their diet in a lasting way. There is no need for an exact nutrition plan for this, as simply avoiding certain foods already has a great health benefit.

The approach of this low-fat diet only affects those who find themselves struggling with an incorrect lifestyle. This means that you will also need to quit smoking and start training. The Dash diet requires eliminating alcohol and sodium chloride (the synthetic salt). But also to drastically reduce the consumption of foods rich in saturated fats, such as red meat, cheeses, packaged products and sweets.

Instead, it promotes the intake of fish (2-6 portions per day) and fresh fruit and vegetables (7-8 portions). In particular, foods rich in potassium, calcium, magnesium and omega 3 fatty acids such as oily nuts. Supplements that support the work of the heart, such as arginine, and low mineral content water (1.5 / 2 l per day) are also allowed.

Do you notice any similarities? In fact it is very reminiscent of the Mediterranean diet, with a few adjustments!

As we have said, the Dash diet aims to improve health by keeping pressure under control: it is useful both in prevention and in case of hypertension problems already present. Potassium, calcium, fiber and protein are considered the fundamental nutrients to ensure that the pressure remains in the right levels but also essential for this diet to keep the sodium content low in the proposed foods. How? Obviously by limiting the salt consumption that is used in the kitchen. As already mentioned, the Dash diet is very similar to the Italian Mediterranean diet in which the consumption of seasonal fruit and vegetables, whole grains, good fats and proteins is preferred, instead limiting saturated fats, salt and all those substances that in some way can damage circulation and heart. However, it is a diet model and has to be customized according to individual needs and can also be used to lose weight.

In addition to improving blood pressure, this diet promotes intestinal transit, thanks to its high fiber content. Calcium, on the other hand, prevents osteoporosis, while essential fatty acids slow down aging. Finally, the reduced intake of sugars and saturated fats keeps type 2 diabetes and atherosclerosis under control.

DASH diet is the abbreviation of Dietary Approaches to Stop Hypertension. The DASH diet is used to live a healthy lifestyle and prevent diseases like high blood pressure, which is known as hypertension. If you want to lower your blood pressure, reduces the risk of heart attacks, you should follow the DASH diet.

The variety of foods rich in nutrients included in the DASH diet will lower your blood pressure and prevent diseases. If you follow the DASH diet, you will see a big difference in your blood pressure in just two weeks.

Besides lowering blood pressure, it will also help to prevent osteoporosis, cancer, diabetes, and strokes.

Recipes

Breakfast

1 Lemon Zucchini Muffins

Preparation time: 10 minutes

Cooking time: 7 minutes

Servings: 1

Ingredients:

All-purpose flour – 2 cups

Sugar – ½ cup

Baking powder – 1 Tbsp.

Salt – ¼ tsp.

Cinnamon – ¼ tsp.

Nutmeg – ¼ tsp.

Shredded zucchini – 1 cup

Nonfat milk – ¾ cup

Olive oil - 2 Tbsp.

Lemon juice – 2 Tbsp.

Egg – 1

Nonstick cooking spray

Directions:

Preheat the oven to 400F. Grease the muffin tins.

Combine sugar, flour, baking powder, salt, cinnamon, and nutmeg in a bowl.

In another bowl, combine zucchini, milk, oil, lemon juice, and egg. Stir well.

Add zucchini mixture to flour mixture. Stir until just combined.

Pour batter into prepared muffin cups.

Bake for 20 minutes and serve.

Nutrition:

Calories: 145

Fat: 4g

Carb: 25g

Protein: 3g

Sodium 62mg

2 Greek-Style Breakfast Scramble

Preparation time: 10 minutes

Cooking time: 8 minutes

Servings: 1

Ingredients:

Nonstick cooking spray

Fresh spinach – 1 cup, chopped

Mushrooms – ½ cup, chopped

Onion – ¼, chopped

Whole egg – 1, and 2 egg whites

Feta cheese – 2 Tbsp.

Freshly ground black pepper to taste

Directions:

Heat a skillet over medium heat.

Spray with cooking spray and add spinach, mushrooms, and onion.

Sauté for 2 to 3 minutes or until onions turn translucent and spinach has wilted

Meanwhile, whisk egg and egg whites together in a bowl.

Add feta cheese and pepper.

Pour egg mixture over vegetables.

Cook eggs, stirring with a spatula, for 3 to 4 minutes, or until eggs are cooked.

Serve.

Nutrition:

Calories: 150

Fat: 7g

Carb: 6g

Protein: 17g

Sodium 440mg

3 Blueberry Green Smoothie

Preparation time: 10 minutes

Cooking time: 0 minutes

Servings: 2

Ingredients:

Chopped mixed greens – 2 cups (such as collard greens, mustard greens, kale, and spinach)

Water – ¼ cup

Chopped carrot – 1/3 cup

Frozen blueberries – ½ cup

Chopped unpeeled cucumber – ½ cup

Unsweetened almond milk – ¼ cup

Ice cubes – 4

Directions:

Place the greens and water in a blender. Blend until smooth. Add the remaining ingredients and blend until desired consistency is achieved.

Serve.

Nutrition:

Calories: 82

Fat: 1g

Carb: 17g

Protein: 4g

Sodium 66mg

4 Green Smoothie

Preparation time: 5 minutes

Cooking time: 0 minutes

Servings: 2

Ingredients:

Spinach – 2 cups

Large kale leaves – 2, chopped

Water – ¾ cup

Frozen banana – 1 large, chopped

Frozen mango – ½ cup

Frozen peach – ½ cup

Ground flaxseeds – 1 Tbsp.

Almond butter – 1 Tbsp.

Directions:

Place the spinach, kale, and water in the blender.

Blend until smooth.

Then add fruit, flaxseeds, and nut butter and blend until smooth.

Serve.

Nutrition:

Calories: 157

Fat: 2g

Carb: 35g

Protein: 5g

Sodium 48mg

5 Fascinating Spinach and Beef Meatballs

Preparation time: 10 minutes

Cooking time: 20 minutes

Servings: 2

Ingredients:

½ cup onion

4 garlic cloves

1 whole egg

¼ teaspoon oregano

Pepper as needed

1 pound lean ground beef

10 ounces spinach

Directions:

Preheat your oven to 375 degrees F.

Take a bowl and mix in the rest of the ingredients, and using your hands, roll into meatballs.

Transfer to a sheet tray and bake for 20 minutes.

Enjoy!

Nutrition:

Calorie: 200

Fat: 8g

Carbohydrates: 5g

Protein: 29g

Sodium 350mg

6 Rosemary Rice

Preparation time: 10 minutes

Cooking time: 2 hours

Servings: 4

Ingredients:

1 cup wild rice

½ cup spring onions, chopped

½ cup cherry tomatoes, halved

2 cups water

1 teaspoon rosemary, dried

A pinch of salt and black pepper

Directions:

1. In your slow cooker, combine the rice with the water and the other ingredients, put the lid on and cook on High for 2 hours.

2. Stir the mix more time, divide it into bowls and serve for breakfast.

Nutrition: Calories 152, Fat .0.6g, Cholesterol 0mg, Sodium 10mg, Carbohydrate 32g, Fiber 3.2g, Sugars 1.9g, Protein 6.3g, Potassium 263mg

7 Almond Quinoa

Preparation time: 10 minutes

Cooking time: 4 hours

Servings: 4

Ingredients:

1 teaspoon vanilla extract

1 cup quinoa

1/8 coconut flakes

¼ cup cranberries

2 teaspoons stevia

3 cups coconut water

1/8 cup almonds, sliced

Directions:

In your slow cooker, mix the coconut water with the quinoa, vanilla, stevia, coconut, almonds and cranberries, cover and cook on Low for 4 hours.

Stir the quinoa mix, divide it between plates and serve for breakfast.

Nutrition: Calories 259, Fat .8.6g, Cholesterol 0mg, Sodium 194mg, Carbohydrate 39.3g, Fiber 6.7g, Sugars 6g, Protein 8.4g, Potassium 768mg

Soup

8 Coconut Avocado Soup

Serving: 4

Preparation time: 5 minutes

Cooking Time: 5-10 minutes

Ingredients:

2 cups vegetable stock

2 teaspoons Thai green curry paste

Pepper as needed

1 avocado, chopped

1 tablespoon cilantro, chopped

Lime wedges

1 cup coconut milk

Directions:

Add milk, avocado, curry paste, pepper to blender and blend.

Take a pan and place it over medium heat.

Add mixture and heat, simmer for 5 minutes.

Stir in seasoning, cilantro and simmer for 1 minute.

Serve and enjoy!

Nutrition:

Calories: 250

Fat: 30g

Net Carbohydrates: 2g

Protein: 4g

9 Coconut Arugula Soup

Serving: 4

Preparation time: 5 minutes

Cooking Time: 5-10 minutes

Ingredients:

Black pepper as needed

1 tablespoon olive oil

2 tablespoons chives, chopped

2 garlic cloves, minced

10 ounces baby arugula

2 tablespoons tarragon, chopped

4 tablespoons coconut milk yogurt

6 cups chicken stock

2 tablespoons mint, chopped

1 onion, chopped

½ cup coconut milk

Directions:

Take a saucepan and place it over medium-high heat, add oil and let it heat up.

Add onion and garlic and fry for 5 minutes.

Stir in stock and reduce the heat, let it simmer.

Stir in tarragon, arugula, mint, parsley and cook for 6 minutes.

Mix in seasoning , chives, coconut yogurt and serve.

Enjoy!

Nutrition:

Calories: 180

Fat: 14g

Net Carbohydrates: 20g

Protein: 2g

10   Awesome Cabbage Soup

Preparation time: 7 minutes

Cooking Time: 25 minutes

Serving: 3

Ingredients:

3 cups non-fat beef stock

2 garlic cloves, minced

1 tablespoon tomato paste

2 cups cabbage, chopped

½ yellow onion

½ cup carrot, chopped

½ cup green beans

½ cup zucchini, chopped

½ teaspoon basil

½ teaspoon oregano

Sunflower seeds and pepper as needed

Directions:

Grease a pot with nonstick cooking spray.

Place it over medium heat and allow the oil to heat up.

Add onions, carrots, and garlic and sauté for 5 minutes.

Add broth, tomato paste, green beans, cabbage, basil, oregano, sunflower seeds, and pepper.

Bring the whole mix to a boil and reduce the heat, simmer for 5-10 minutes until all veggies are tender.

Add zucchini and simmer for 5 minutes more.

Sever hot and enjoy!

Nutrition:

Calories: 22

Fat: 0g

Carbohydrates: 5g

Protein: 1g

11   Ginger Zucchini Avocado Soup

Preparation time: 7 minutes

Cooking Time: 25 minutes

Serving: 3

Ingredients:

1 red bell pepper, chopped

1 big avocado

1 teaspoon ginger, grated

Pepper as needed

2 tablespoons avocado oil

4 scallions, chopped

1 tablespoon lemon juice

29 ounces vegetable stock

1 garlic clove, minced

2 zucchini, chopped

1 cup water

Directions:

Take a pan and place over medium heat, add onion and fry for 3 minutes.

Stir in ginger, garlic and cook for 1 minute.

Mix in seasoning, zucchini stock, water and boil for 10 minutes.

Remove soup from fire and let it sit, blend in avocado and blend using an immersion blender.

Heat over low heat for a while.

Adjust your seasoning and add lemon juice, bell pepper.

Serve and enjoy!

Nutrition:

Calories: 155

Fat: 11g

Carbohydrates: 10g

Protein: 7g

12   Greek Lemon and Chicken Soup

Preparation time: 15 minutes

Cooking Time: 30 minutes

Serving: 3

Ingredients:

2 cups cooked chicken, chopped

2 medium carrots, chopped

½ cup onion, chopped

¼ cup lemon juice

1 clove garlic, minced

1 can cream of chicken soup, fat-free and low sodium

2 cans chicken broth, fat-free

¼ teaspoon ground black pepper

2/3 cup long-grain rice

2 tablespoons parsley, snipped

Directions:

Add all of the listed ingredients to a pot (except rice and parsley).

Season with sunflower seeds and pepper.

Bring the mix to a boil over medium-high heat.

Stir in rice and set heat to medium.

Simmer for 20 minutes until rice is tender.

Garnish parsley and enjoy!

Nutrition:

Calories: 582

Fat: 33g

Carbohydrates: 35g

Protein: 32g

Meat

13   Pork And Sweet Potatoes with Chili

Preparation time: 10 minutes

Cooking time: 1 hour and 20 minutes

Servings: 8

Ingredients:

2 pounds sweet potatoes, chopped

A drizzle of olive oil

1 yellow onion, chopped

2 pounds pork meat, ground

1 tablespoon chili powder

Black pepper to the taste

1 teaspoon cumin, ground

½ teaspoon garlic powder

½ teaspoon oregano, chopped

½ teaspoon cinnamon powder

1 cup low-sodium veggie stock

½ cup cilantro, chopped

Directions:

Heat up the a pan with the oil over medium-high heat, add sweet potatoes and onion, stir, cook for 15 minutes and transfer to a bowl.

Heat up the pan again over medium-high heat, add pork, stir and brown for 5 minutes.

Add black pepper, cumin, garlic powder, oregano, chili powder, cinnamon, stock, return potatoes and onion, stir and cook for 1 hour over medium heat.

Add the cilantro, toss, divide into bowls and serve.

Enjoy!

Nutrition: calories 320, fat 7, fiber 6, carbs 12, protein 22

14   Pork And Pumpkin Chili

Preparation time: 10 minutes

Cooking time: 1 hour and 30 minutes

Servings: 6

Ingredients:

1 green bell pepper, chopped

2 cups yellow onion, chopped

1 tablespoon olive oil

6 garlic cloves, minced

28 ounces canned tomatoes, no-salt-added and chopped

1 and ½ pounds pork, ground

6 ounces low-sodium tomato paste

14 ounces pumpkin puree

1 cup low-sodium chicken stock

2 and ½ teaspoons oregano, dried

1 and ½ teaspoon cinnamon, ground

1 and ½ tablespoon chili powder

Black pepper to the taste

Directions:

Heat up a pot with the oil over medium-high heat, add bell peppers and onion, stir and cook for 7 minutes.

Add garlic and the pork, toss and cook for 10 minutes.

Add tomatoes, tomato paste, pumpkin puree, stock, oregano, cinnamon, chili powder and pepper, stir, cover, cook over medium heat for 1 hour and 10 minutes, divide into bowls and serve.

Enjoy!

Nutrition: calories 289, fat 12, fiber 8, carbs 12, protein 20

15   Spiced Pork Soup

Preparation time: 10 minutes

Cooking time: 1 hour and 30 minutes

Servings: 6

Ingredients:

3 carrots, chopped

1 pound pork meat, cubed

1 tomato, chopped

3 mushrooms, sliced

6 star anise

4 bay leaves

5 ginger slices

2 tablespoons Sichuan peppercorns

1 an ½ tablespoons fennel powder

1 teaspoon coriander, ground

1 tablespoon cumin powder

¼ teaspoon five spice powder

Black pepper to the taste

A bunch of scallions, chopped

8 cups water

1/3 cup coconut aminos

Directions:

Put the water in a pot and heat up over medium heat.

Add carrots, pork, tomato, mushrooms, star anise, bay leaves, ginger, peppercorns, fennel, coriander, cumin, five spice, black pepper, aminos and scallions, stir, bring to a boil and cook for 1 hour and 30 minutes.

Discard star anise, ginger, bay leaves and peppercorns, ladle the soup into bowls and serve.

Enjoy!

Nutrition: calories 250, fat 2, fiber 7, carbs 14, protein 14

16   Ground Pork And Kale Soup

Preparation time: 10 minutes

Cooking time: 30 minutes

Servings: 4

Ingredients:

1 pound pork, ground

3 carrots, chopped

4 potatoes, chopped

1 yellow onion, chopped

½ bunch kale, chopped

4 garlic cloves, minced

2 cups squash, cooked and pureed

2 quarts low-sodium veggie stock

Black pepper to the taste

3 teaspoons Italian seasoning

Directions:

Heat up a pot over medium-high heat, add pork, stir, brown for 5 minutes and transfer to a bowl.

Heat up the pot again over medium heat, add potatoes, onion, carrots, kale, garlic and pepper, stir and cook for 10 minutes. Return beef, also add stock, squash puree and Italian seasoning, stir, simmer over medium heat for 15 minutes, ladle into bowls and serve.

Enjoy!

Nutrition: calories 270, fat 12, fiber 6, carbs 12, protein 23

17   Peaches and Kale Steak Salad

Preparation time: 10 minutes

Cooking time: 12 minutes

Servings: 2

Ingredients:

2 peaches, chopped

3 handfuls kale, chopped

8 ounces pork steak, cut into strips

1 tablespoon avocado oil

A drizzle of olive oil

1 tablespoon balsamic vinegar

Directions:

Heat up a pan with the avocado oil over medium-high heat, add steak strips, cook them for 6 minutes on each side and transfer to a salad bowl.

Add peaches, kale, olive oil and vinegar, toss and serve.

Enjoy!

Nutrition: calories 240, fat 5, fiber 4, carbs 8, protein 15

18   Garlic Pork Meatballs

Preparation Time: 10 minutes

Cooking Time: 28 minutes

Servings: 2

Ingredients:

2 pork medallions

1 teaspoon minced garlic

¼ cup of coconut milk

1 tablespoon olive oil

1 teaspoon cayenne pepper

Directions:

Sprinkle each pork medallion with cayenne pepper.

Heat up olive oil in the skillet and add meat.

Roast the pork medallions for 3 minutes from each side.

After this, add coconut milk and minced garlic. Close the lid and simmer the meat for 20 minutes on low heat.

Nutrition:

284 calories,

25.9g protein,

2.6g carbohydrates,

18.8g fat,

0.9g fiber,

70mg cholesterol,

60mg sodium,

103mg potassium.

Seafood

19   Creamy Salmon and Asparagus Mix

Preparation time: 10 minutes

Cooking time: 10 minutes

Servings: 6

Ingredients:

1 tablespoon lemon zest, grated

1 tablespoon lemon juice

Black pepper to the taste

1 cup coconut cream

1 pound asparagus, trimmed

20 ounces salmon, skinless and boneless

1-ounce parmesan cheese, grated

Directions:

Put some water in a pot, add a pinch of salt, bring to a boil over medium heat, add asparagus, cook for 1 minute, transfer to a bowl filled with ice water, drain and put in a bowl.

Heat up the pot with the water again over medium heat, add salmon, cook for 5 minutes and also drain.

In a bowl, mix lemon peel with cream and lemon juice and whisk

Heat up a pan over medium-high heat, asparagus, cream and pepper, cook for 1 more minute, divide between plates, add salmon and serve with grated parmesan.

Enjoy!

Nutrition: calories 354, fat 2, fiber 2, carbs 2, protein 4

20   Salmon And Brussels Sprouts

Preparation time: 10 minutes

Cooking time: 20 minutes

Servings: 6

Ingredients:

2 tablespoons brown sugar

1 teaspoon onion powder

1 teaspoon garlic powder

1 teaspoon smoked paprika

3 tablespoons olive oil

1 and ¼ pounds Brussels sprouts, halved

6 medium salmon fillets, boneless

Directions:

In a bowl, mix sugar with onion powder, garlic powder, smoked paprika and 2 tablespoon olive oil and whisk well.

Spread Brussels sprouts on a lined baking sheet, drizzle the rest of the olive oil, toss to coat, introduce in the oven at 450 degrees F and bake for 5 minutes.

Add salmon fillets brush with sugar mix you've prepared, introduce in the oven and bake for 15 minutes more.

Divide everything between plates and serve.

Enjoy!

Nutrition: calories 212, fat 5, fiber 3, carbs 12, protein 8

21   Salmon and Beets Mix

Preparation time: 10 minutes

Cooking time: 35 minutes

Servings: 4

Ingredients:

1-pound medium beets, sliced

6 tablespoons olive oil

1 and ½ pounds salmon fillets, skinless and boneless

Black pepper to the taste

1 tablespoon chives, chopped

1 tablespoon parsley, chopped

3 tablespoon shallots, chopped

1 tablespoon lemon zest, grated

¼ cup lemon juice

Directions:

In a bowl, mix beets with ½ tablespoon oil and toss to coat, season with black pepper, spread on a lined baking sheet and bake in the oven at 450 degrees F for 20 minutes.

Add salmon, brush it with the rest of the oil, introduce in the oven and bake for 15 minutes more.

In a bowl, combine the chives with the parsley, shallots, lemon zest and lemon juice and toss.

Divide the salmon and the beets between plates, drizzle the chives mix on top and serve.

Enjoy!

Nutrition: calories 272, fat 6, fiber 2, carbs 12, protein 9

22   Garlic Shrimp Mix

Preparation time: 10 minutes

Cooking time: 10 minutes

Servings: 4

Ingredients:

1 pound shrimp, deveined and peeled

2 teaspoons olive oil

6 tablespoons lemon juice

3 tablespoons dill, chopped

1 tablespoon oregano, chopped

2 garlic cloves, chopped

Black pepper to the taste

¾ cup non-fat yogurt

½ pounds cherry tomatoes, halved

Directions:

Heat up a pan with the oil over medium-high heat, add the shrimp and cook for 3 minutes.

Add lemon juice, dill, oregano, garlic, black pepper, yogurt and tomatoes, toss, cook for 5 minutes more, divide into bowls and serve.

Enjoy!

Nutrition: calories 253, fat 6, fiber 6, carbs 10, protein 17

Vegetarian and Vegan

23   Eggplant Parmesan Stacks

Preparation time: 15 minutes

Cooking time: 20 minutes

Servings: 4

Ingredients:

1 large eggplant, cut into thick slices

2 tablespoons olive oil, divided

¼ teaspoon kosher or sea salt

¼ teaspoon ground black pepper

1 cup panko bread crumbs

¼ cup freshly grated Parmesan cheese

5 to 6 garlic cloves, minced

½ pound fresh mozzarella, sliced

1½ cups lower-sodium marinara

½ cup fresh basil leaves, torn

Directions:

Preheat the oven to 425°F. Coat the eggplant slices in 1 tablespoon olive oil and sprinkle with the salt and black pepper. Put on a large baking sheet, then roast for 10 to 12 minutes, until soft with crispy edges. Remove the eggplant and set the oven to a low broil.

In a bowl, stir the remaining tablespoon of olive oil, bread crumbs, Parmesan cheese, and garlic. Remove the cooled eggplant from the baking sheet and clean it.

Create layers on the same baking sheet by stacking a roasted eggplant slice with a slice of mozzarella, a tablespoon of marinara, and a tablespoon of the bread crumb mixture, repeating with 2 layers of each ingredient. Cook under the broiler within 3 to 4 minutes until the cheese is melted and bubbly.

Nutrition: Calories: 377 Fat: 22g Sodium: 509mg Carbohydrate: 29g Protein: 16g

24   Roasted Vegetable Enchiladas

Preparation time: 15 minutes

Cooking time: 45 minutes

Servings: 8

Ingredients:

2 zucchinis, diced

1 red bell pepper, seeded and sliced

1 red onion, peeled and sliced

2 ears corn

2 tablespoons canola oil

1 can no-salt-added black beans, drained

1½ tablespoons chili powder

2 teaspoon ground cumin

1/8 teaspoon kosher or sea salt

½ teaspoon ground black pepper

8 (8-inch) whole-wheat tortillas

1 cup Enchilada Sauce or store-bought enchilada sauce

½ cup shredded Mexican-style cheese

½ cup plain nonfat Greek yogurt

½ cup cilantro leaves, chopped

Directions:

Preheat oven to 400°F. Place the zucchini, red bell pepper, and red onion on a baking sheet. Place the ears of corn separately on the same baking sheet. Drizzle all with the canola oil and toss to coat. Roast for 10 to 12 minutes, until the vegetables are tender. Remove and reduce the temperature to 375°F.

Cut the corn from the cob. Transfer the corn kernels, zucchini, red bell pepper, and onion to a bowl and stir in the black beans, chili powder, cumin, salt, and black pepper until combined.

Oiled a 9-by-13-inch baking dish with cooking spray. Line up the tortillas in the greased baking dish. Evenly distribute the vegetable bean filling into each tortilla. Pour half of the enchilada sauce and sprinkle half of the shredded cheese on top of the filling.

Roll each tortilla into enchilada shape and place them seam-side down. Pour the remaining enchilada sauce and sprinkle the remaining cheese over the enchiladas. Bake for 25 minutes until the cheese is melted and bubbly. Serve the enchiladas with Greek yogurt and chopped cilantro.

Nutrition: Calories: 335 Fat: 15g Sodium: 557mg Carbohydrate: 42g Protein: 13g

25   Lentil Avocado Tacos

Preparation time: 15 minutes

Cooking time: 35 minutes

Servings: 6

Ingredients:

1 tablespoon canola oil

½ yellow onion, peeled and diced

2-3 garlic cloves, minced

1½ cups dried lentils

½ teaspoon kosher or sea salt

3 to 3½ cups unsalted vegetable or chicken stock

2½ tablespoons Taco Seasoning or store-bought low-sodium taco seasoning

16 (6-inch) corn tortillas, toasted

2 ripe avocados, peeled and sliced

Directions:

Heat-up the canola oil in a large skillet or Dutch oven over medium heat. Cook the onion within 4 to 5 minutes, until soft. Mix in the garlic and cook within 30 seconds until fragrant. Then add the lentils, salt, and stock. Bring to a simmer for 25 to 35 minutes, adding additional stock if needed.

When there's only a small amount of liquid left in the pan, and the lentils are al dente, stir in the taco seasoning and let simmer for 1 to 2 minutes. Taste and adjust the seasoning, if necessary. Spoon the lentil mixture into tortillas and serve with the avocado slices.

Nutrition: Calories: 400 Fat: 14g Sodium: 336mg Carbohydrate: 64g Fiber: 15g Protein: 16g

26 Tomato & Olive Orecchiette with Basil Pesto

Preparation time: 15 minutes

Cooking time: 25 minutes

Servings: 6

Ingredients:

12 ounces orecchiette pasta

2 tablespoons olive oil

1-pint cherry tomatoes, quartered

½ cup Basil Pesto or store-bought pesto

¼ cup kalamata olives, sliced

1 tablespoon dried oregano leaves

¼ teaspoon kosher or sea salt

½ teaspoon freshly cracked black pepper

¼ teaspoon crushed red pepper flakes

2 tablespoons freshly grated Parmesan cheese

Directions:

Boil a large pot of water. Cook the orecchiette, drain and transfer the pasta to a large nonstick skillet.

Put the skillet over medium-low heat, then heat the olive oil. Stir in the cherry tomatoes, pesto, olives, oregano, salt, black pepper, and crushed red pepper flakes. Cook within 8 to 10 minutes, until heated throughout. Serve the pasta with the freshly grated Parmesan cheese.

Nutrition: Calories: 332 Fat: 13g Sodium: 389mg Carbohydrate: 44g Protein: 9g

27 Italian Stuffed Portobello Mushroom Burgers

Preparation time: 15 minutes

Cooking time: 25 minutes

Servings: 4

Ingredients:

1 tablespoon olive oil

4 large portobello mushrooms, washed and dried

½ yellow onion, peeled and diced

4 garlic cloves, peeled and minced

1 can cannellini beans, drained

½ cup fresh basil leaves, torn

½ cup panko bread crumbs

1/8 teaspoon kosher or sea salt

¼ teaspoon ground black pepper

1 cup lower-sodium marinara, divided

½ cup shredded mozzarella cheese

4 whole-wheat buns, toasted

1 cup fresh arugula

Directions:

Heat-up the olive oil in a large skillet to medium-high heat. Sear the mushrooms for 4 to 5 minutes per side, until slightly soft. Place on a baking sheet. Preheat the oven to a low broil. Put the onion in the skillet and cook for 4 to 5 minutes, until slightly soft. Mix in the garlic then cooks within 30 to 60 seconds. Move the onions plus garlic to a bowl. Add the cannellini beans and smash with the back of a fork to form a chunky paste. Stir in the basil, bread crumbs, salt, and black pepper and half of the marinara. Cook for 5 minutes.

Remove the bean mixture from the stove and divide among the mushroom caps. Spoon the remaining marinara over the stuffed mushrooms and top each with the mozzarella cheese. Broil within 3 to 4 minutes, until the cheese is melted and bubbly. Transfer the burgers to the toasted whole-wheat buns and top with the arugula.

Nutrition: Calories: 407 Fat: 9g Sodium: 575mg Carbohydrate: 63g Protein: 25g

---

Side Dishes, Salads & Appetizers

28   Baby Spinach And Grains Mix

Preparation time: 10 minutes

Cooking time: 4 hours

Servings: 12

Ingredients:

1 butternut squash, peeled and cubed

1 cup whole grain blend, uncooked

12 ounces low-sodium veggie stock

6 ounces baby spinach

1 yellow onion, chopped

3 garlic cloves, minced

1/2 cup water

2 teaspoons thyme, chopped

A pinch of black pepper

Directions:

In your slow cooker, mix the squash with whole grain, onion, garlic, water, thyme, black pepper, stock and spinach, cover and cook on Low for 4 hours.

Divide between plates and serve as a side dish.

Nutrition: Calories78, Fat 0.6g, Cholesterol 0mg, Sodium 259mg, Carbohydrate 16.4g, Fiber 1.8g, Sugars 2g, Protein 2.5g, Potassium 138mg

29   Italians Style Mushroom Mix

Preparation time: 10 minutes

Cooking time: 4 hours

Servings: 6

Ingredients:

1 pound mushrooms, halved

1 teaspoon Italian seasoning

3 tablespoons olive oil

1 cup tomato sauce, no-salt-added

1 yellow onion, chopped

Directions:

In your slow cooker, mix the mushrooms with the oil, onion, Italian seasoning and tomato sauce, toss, cover and cook on Low for 4 hours.

Divide between plates and serve as a side dish.

Nutrition: Calories96, Fat 7.5g, Cholesterol 1mg, Sodium 219mg, Carbohydrate 6.5g, Fiber 1.8g, Sugars 3.9g, Protein 3.1g, Potassium 403mg

30   Spicy Brussels Sprouts

Preparation time: 10 minutes

Cooking time: 20 minutes

Servings: 6

Ingredients:

2 pounds Brussels sprouts, halved

2 tablespoons olive oil

A pinch of black pepper

1 tablespoon sesame oil

2 garlic cloves, minced

½ cup coconut aminos

2 teaspoons apple cider vinegar

1 tablespoon coconut sugar

2 teaspoons chili sauce

A pinch of red pepper flakes

Sesame seeds for serving

Directions:

Spread the sprouts on a lined baking dish, add the olive oil, the sesame oil, black pepper, garlic, aminos, vinegar, coconut sugar, chili sauce and pepper flakes, toss well, introduce in the oven and bake at 425 degrees F for 20 minutes.

Divide the sprouts between plates, sprinkle sesame seeds on top and serve as a side dish.

Enjoy!

Nutrition: calories 176, fat 3, fiber 6, carbs 14, protein 9

31   Pasta with Tomatoes and Peas

Preparation Time: 10 minutes

Cooking Time: 15 minutes

Servings: 2

Ingredients

½ cup whole-grain pasta of choice

8 cups water, plus ¼ for finishing

1 cup frozen peas

1 tablespoon olive oil

1 cup cherry tomatoes, halved

¼ teaspoon freshly ground black pepper

1 teaspoon dried basil

¼ cup grated Parmesan cheese (low-sodium)

Directions

1. Cook the pasta al dente.

2. Add the water to the same pot you used to cook the pasta. Bring the water to a boil and add the peas. Cook until tender, but still firm (about 5 minutes). Drain and set aside.

3. Heat the oil in a large skillet over medium heat. Add the cherry tomatoes. Put a lid on the skillet and let the tomatoes soften for about 5 minutes, stirring a few times.

4. Season with black pepper and basil.

5. Toss in the pasta, peas, and ¼ cup of water. Stir and remove from the heat.

6. Serve topped with Parmesan cheese.

Nutrition: Total Calories: 266; Total Fat: 12g; Saturated Fat: 4g; Cholesterol: 10mg; Sodium: 320mg; Potassium: 313mg; Total Carbohydrates: 30g; Fiber: 6g; Sugars: 5g; Protein: 13g

32   Healthy Vegetable Fried Rice

Preparation Time: 5 minutes

Cooking Time: 10 minutes

Servings: 4

Ingredients

For The Sauce:

⅓ cup garlic vinegar

1½ tablespoons dark molasses

1 teaspoon onion powder

For The Fried Rice:

1 teaspoon olive oil

2 whole eggs plus 4 egg whites, lightly beaten

1 cup frozen mixed vegetables

1 cup frozen edamame

2 cups cooked brown rice

Directions

To make the sauce

Prepare the sauce by combining the garlic vinegar, molasses, and onion powder in a glass jar. Shake well.

To make the fried rice

1. Heat oil in a large wok or skillet over medium-high heat. Add eggs and egg whites and let cook until the eggs are set (about 1 minute). Break eggs into small pieces with a spatula or. Add frozen mixed vegetables and frozen edamame. Cook for 4 minutes, stirring frequently.

2. Add the brown rice and sauce to the vegetable-and-egg mixture. Cook for 5 minutes or until heated through.

3. Serve immediately.

Nutrition: Total Calories: 210; Total Fat: 6g; Saturated Fat: 1g; Cholesterol: 93mg; Sodium: 113mg; Potassium: 183mg; Total Carbohydrates: 28g; Fiber: 3g; Sugars: 6g; Protein: 13g

33   Portobello-Mushroom Cheeseburgers

Preparation Time: 5 minutes

Cooking Time: 10 minutes

Servings: 4

Ingredients

4 Portobello mushrooms, caps removed and brushed clean

1 tablespoon olive oil

½ teaspoon freshly ground black pepper

1 tablespoon red wine vinegar

4 slices reduced-fat Swiss cheese, sliced thin

4 whole-wheat 100-calorie sandwich thins

½ avocado, sliced thin

Directions

1. Heat a skillet or grill pan over medium-high heat. Clean the mushrooms and remove the stems. Brush each cap with olive oil and sprinkle with black pepper. Place in skillet, cap-side up and cook for about 4 minutes. Flip and cook for another 4 minutes.

2. Sprinkle with the red wine vinegar and turn over. Add the cheese and cook for 2 more minutes. For optimal melting, place a lid loosely over the pan.

3. Toast the sandwich thins. Create your burgers by topping each with sliced avocado.

4. Enjoy immediately.

Nutrition: Total Calories: 245; Total Fat: 12g; Saturated Fat: 3g; Cholesterol: 15mg; Sodium: 266mg; Potassium: 507mg; Total Carbohydrates: 28g; Fiber: 8g; Sugars: 4g; Protein: 14g

34   Baked Chickpea-and-Rosemary Omelet

Preparation Time: 10 minutes

Cooking Time: 15 minutes

Servings: 2

Ingredients

½ tablespoon olive oil

4 eggs

¼ cup grated Parmesan cheese

1 (15-ounce) can chickpeas, drained and rinsed

2 cups packed baby spinach

1 cup button mushrooms, chopped

2 sprigs rosemary, leaves picked (or 2 teaspoons dried rosemary)

Salt

Freshly ground black pepper

Directions

1. Preheat the oven to 400°F and place a baking tray on the middle shelf.

2. Line an 8-inch springform pan with baking paper and grease generously with olive oil. If you don't have a springform pan, grease an oven-safe skillet (or cast-iron skillet) with olive oil.

3. Lightly whisk together the eggs and Parmesan.

4. Place chickpeas in the pan. Layer the spinach and mushrooms on top of the beans. Pour the egg mixture on top and scatter the rosemary. Season to taste with salt and pepper.

5. Place the pan on the preheated tray and bake until golden and puffy and the center feels firm and springy (about 15 minutes).

6. Remove from the oven, slice, and serve immediately.

Nutrition: Total Calories: 418; Total Fat: 19g; Saturated Fat: 6g; Cholesterol: 382mg; Sodium: 595mg; Potassium: 273mg; Total Carbohydrates: 33g; Fiber: 12g; Sugars: 2g; Protein: 30g

35   Easy Chickpea Veggie Burgers

Preparation Time: 10 minutes

Cooking Time: 20 minutes

Servings: 4

Ingredients

1 15-ounce can chickpeas, drained and rinsed

½ cup frozen spinach, thawed

⅓ cup rolled oats

1 teaspoon garlic powder

1 teaspoon onion powder

Directions 1. Preheat oven to 400°F. Grease a sheet or line one with parchment paper and set aside.

2. In a mixing bowl, add half of the beans and mash with a fork until fairly smooth. Set aside.

3. Add the remaining half of the beans, spinach, oats, and spices to a food processor or blender and blend until puréed. Add the mixture to the bowl of mashed beans and stir until well combined.

4. Divide mixture into 4 equal portions and shape into patties. Bake for 7 to 10 minutes. Carefully turn over and bake for another 7 to 10 minutes or until crusty on the outside.

5. Place on a whole grain bun with your favorite toppings.

Nutrition: Total Calories: 118; Total Fat: 1g; Saturated Fat: 0g; Cholesterol: 7mg; Sodium: 108mg; Potassium: 83mg; Total Carbohydrates: 21g; Fiber: 7g; Sugars: 0g; Protein: 7g

36   Watercress Salad

Preparation Time: 10 minutes

Cooking Time: 4 minutes

Servings: 2

Ingredients:

2 cups asparagus, chopped

16 ounces shrimp, cooked

4 cups watercress, torn

1 tablespoon apple cider vinegar

¼ cup olive oil

Directions:

In the mixing bowl mix up asparagus, shrimps, watercress, and olive oil.

Nutrition:

264 calories,

28.3g protein,

4.5g carbohydrates,

14.8g fat,

1.8g fiber,

239mg cholesterol,

300mg sodium,

393mg potassium.

37   Seafood Arugula Salad

Preparation Time: 5 minutes

Cooking Time: 10 minutes

Servings: 2

Ingredients:

1 tablespoon olive oil

2 cups shrimps, cooked

1 cup arugula

1 tablespoon cilantro, chopped

Directions:

Put all ingredients in the salad bowl and shake well.

Nutrition:

61 calories,

6.6g protein,

0.2g carbohydrates,

3.7g fat,

0.1g fiber,

123mg cholesterol,

216mg sodium,

20mg potassium

Dessert and Snacks

38   Summer Jam

Preparation time: 10 minutes

Cooking time: 3 hours

Servings: 6

Ingredients:

2 cups coconut sugar

4 cups cherries, pitted

2 tablespoons lemon juice

3 tablespoons gelatin

Directions:

In your slow cooker, mix lemon juice with gelatin, cherries and coconut sugar, stir, cover, cook on High for 3 hours, divide into bowls and serve cold.

Nutrition Calories 171, Fat 0.1g, Cholesterol 0mg, Sodium 41mg, Carbohydrate 37.2g, Fiber 0.7g, Sugars 0.1g, Protein 3.8g, Potassium 122mg

39   Cinnamon Pudding

Preparation time: 10 minutes

Cooking time: 5 hours

Servings: 4

Ingredients:

2 cups white rice

1 cup coconut sugar

2 cinnamon sticks

6 and ½ cups water

½ cup coconut, shredded

Directions:

In your slow cooker, mix water with the rice, sugar, cinnamon and coconut, stir, cover, cook on High for 5 hours, discard cinnamon, divide pudding into bowls and serve warm.

Nutrition: Calories 400, Fat 4g, Cholesterol 0mg, Sodium 28mg, Carbohydrate 81.2g, Fiber 2.7g, Sugars 0.8g, Protein 7.2g, Potassium 151mg

40   Orange Compote

Preparation time: 10 minutes

Cooking time: 2 hours and 30 minutes

Servings: 4

Ingredients:

½ pound oranges, peeled and cut into segments

½ pound plums, pitted and halved

1 cup orange juice

3 tablespoons coconut sugar

½ cup water

Directions:

In the slow cooker, combine the oranges with the plums, orange juice and the other ingredients, put the lid on and cook on High for 2 hours and 30 minutes.

Stir, divide into bowls and serve cold.

Nutrition: Calories 130, Fat 0.2g, Cholesterol 0mg, Sodium 31mg, Carbohydrate 28.4g, Fiber 1.6g, Sugars 11.4g, Protein 1.8g, Potassium 240mg

41   Chocolate Bars

Preparation time: 10 minutes

Cooking time: 2 hours and 30 minutes

Servings: 12

Ingredients:

1 cup coconut sugar

½ cup dark chocolate chips

1 egg white

¼ cup coconut oil, melted

½ teaspoon vanilla extract

1 teaspoon baking powder

1 and ½ cups almond meal

Directions:

In a bowl, mix the oil with sugar, vanilla extract, egg white, baking powder and almond flour and whisk well

Fold in chocolate chips and stir gently.

Line your slow cooker with parchment paper, grease it, add cookie mix, press on the bottom, cover and cook on low for 2 hours and 30 minutes.

Take cookie sheet out of the slow cooker, cut into medium bars and serve.

Nutrition: Calories 141, Fat 11.8g, Cholesterol 0mg, Sodium 7mg, Carbohydrate 7.7g, Fiber 1.5g, Sugars 3.2g, Protein 3.2g, Potassium 134mg

42   Lemon Zest Pudding

Preparation time: 10 minutes

Cooking time: 5 hours

Servings: 4

Ingredients:

1 cup pineapple juice, natural

Cooking spray

1 teaspoon baking powder

1 cup coconut flour

3 tablespoons avocado oil

3 tablespoons stevia

½ cup pineapple, chopped

½ cup lemon zest, grated

½ cup coconut milk

½ cup pecans, chopped

Directions:

Spray your slow cooker with cooking spray.

In a bowl, mix flour with stevia, baking powder, oil, milk, pecans, pineapple, lemon zest and pineapple juice, stir well, pour into your slow cooker greased with cooking spray, cover and cook on Low for 5 hours.

Divide into bowls and serve.

Nutrition: Calories 431, Fat 29.7g, Cholesterol 0mg, Sodium 8mg, Carbohydrate 47.1g, Fiber 17g, Sugars 10.9g, Protein 8.1g, Potassium 482mg

43   Coconut Figs

Preparation time: 6 minutes

Cooking time: 5 minutes

Servings: 4

Ingredients:

2 tablespoons coconut butter

12 figs, halved

¼ cup coconut sugar

1 cup almonds, toasted and chopped

Directions:

Put butter in a pot, heat up over medium heat, add sugar, whisk well, also add almonds and figs, toss, cook for 5 minutes, divide into small cups and serve cold.

Enjoy!

Nutrition: calories 150, fat 4, fiber 5, carbs 7, protein 4

44   Lemony Banana Mix

Preparation time: 10 minutes

Cooking time: 0 minutes

Servings: 4

Ingredients:

4 bananas, peeled and chopped

5 strawberries, halved

Juice of 2 lemons

4 tablespoons coconut sugar

Directions:

In a bowl, combine the bananas with the strawberries, lemon juice and sugar, toss and serve cold.

Enjoy!

Nutrition: calories 172, fat 7, fiber 5, carbs 5, protein 5

45   Cocoa Banana Dessert Smoothie

Preparation time: 5 minutes

Cooking time: 0 minutes

Servings: 2

Ingredients:

2 medium bananas, peeled

2 teaspoons cocoa powder

½ big avocado, pitted, peeled and mashed

¾ cup almond milk

Directions:

In your blender, combine the bananas with the cocoa, avocado and milk, pulse well, divide into 2 glasses and serve.

Enjoy!

Nutrition: calories 155, fat 3, fiber 4, carbs 6, protein 5

46   Kiwi Bars

Preparation time: 30 minutes

Cooking time: 0 minutes

Servings: 4

Ingredients:

1 cup olive oil

1 and ½ bananas, peeled and chopped

1/3 cup coconut sugar

¼ cup lemon juice

1 teaspoon lemon zest, grated

3 kiwis, peeled and chopped

Directions:

In your food processor, mix bananas with kiwis, almost all the oil, sugar, lemon juice and lemon zest and pulse well.

Grease a pan with the remaining oil, pour the kiwi mix, spread, keep in the fridge for 30 minutes, slice and serve,

Enjoy!

Nutrition: calories 207, fat 3, fiber 3, carbs 4, protein 4

47   Black Tea Bars

Preparation time: 10 minutes

Cooking time: 35 minutes

Servings: 12

Ingredients:

6 tablespoons black tea powder

2 cups almond milk

½ cup low-fat butter

2 cups coconut sugar

4 eggs

2 teaspoons vanilla extract

½ cup olive oil

3 and ½ cups whole wheat flour

1 teaspoon baking soda

3 teaspoons baking powder

Directions:

Put the milk in a pot, heat it up over medium heat, add tea, stir, take off heat and cool down.

Add butter, sugar, eggs, vanilla, oil, flour, baking soda and baking powder, stir well, pour into a square pan, spread, introduce in the oven, bake at 350 degrees F for 35 minutes, cool down, slice and serve. Enjoy!

Nutrition: calories 220, fat 4, fiber 4, carbs 12, protein 7

48   Green Pudding

Preparation time: 2 hours

Cooking time: 5 minutes

Servings: 6

Ingredients:

14 ounces almond milk

2 tablespoons green tea powder

14 ounces coconut cream

3 tablespoons coconut sugar

1 teaspoon gelatin powder

Directions:

Put the milk in a pan, add sugar, gelatin, coconut cream and green tea powder, stir, bring to a simmer, cook for 5 minutes, divide into cups and keep in the fridge for 2 hours before serving.

Enjoy!

Nutrition: calories 170, fat 3, fiber 3, carbs 7, protein 4

49   Lemony Plum Cake

Preparation time: 1 hour and 20 minutes

Cooking time: 40 minutes

Servings: 8

Ingredients:

7 ounces whole wheat flour

1 teaspoon baking powder

1-ounce low-fat butter, soft

1 egg, whisked

5 tablespoons coconut sugar

3 ounces warm almond milk

1 and ¾ pounds plums, pitted and cut into quarters

Zest of 1 lemon, grated

1-ounce almond flakes

Directions:

In a bowl, combine the flour with baking powder, butter, egg, sugar, milk and lemon zest, stir well, transfer dough to a lined cake pan, spread plums and almond flakes all over, introduce in the oven and bake at 350 degrees F for 40 minutes.

Slice and serve cold.

Enjoy

Nutrition: calories 222, fat 4, fiber 2, carbs 7, protein 7

50   Lentils Sweet Bars

Preparation time: 10 minutes

Cooking time: 25 minutes

Servings: 14

Ingredients:

1 cup lentils, cooked, drained and rinsed

1 teaspoon cinnamon powder

2 cups whole wheat flour

1 teaspoon baking powder

½ teaspoon nutmeg, ground

1 cup low-fat butter

1 cup coconut sugar

1 egg

2 teaspoons almond extract

1 cup raisins

2 cups coconut, unsweetened and shredded

Directions:

Put the lentils in a bowl, mash them well using a fork, add cinnamon, flour, baking powder, nutmeg, butter, sugar, egg, almond extract, raisins and coconut, stir, spread on a lined baking sheet, introduce in the oven, bake at 350 degrees F for 25 minutes, cut into bars and serve cold.

Enjoy!

Nutrition: calories 214, fat 4, fiber 2, carbs 5, protein 7

Conclusion

Thank you for reading the DASH Diet – Mediterranean solution! We hope that you have found this book entertaining and most of all informative. Remember that good health is a lifelong process and a journey. Don't despair when you slip up on occasion, just climb back on board.

The DASH diet is based on a pyramid, with the most frequently consumed items as the base. That would be fruits and vegetables. These items are supposed to be consumed liberally, in servings of 8-10 per day, with 4-5 servings of vegetables and 4-5 servings of fruits. Next, 6-8 servings of whole grains are to be eaten daily. While 2-3 servings of dairy are to be consumed per day, meat is eaten in relative moderation. Only lean cuts of skinless poultry and fish are eaten regularly in 3-4 ounce portions. Oils are allowed only in tiny amounts, and nuts with at most 1 serving per day.

The DASH diet was originally developed in the early 1990s. Back then, ideas about the role of fat in the diet were quite different than they are today. In those times it was believed that fat was the cause of heart disease and stroke, and so doctors sought to promote very low-fat diets. Since that time, however, doctors have learned that the role of fat in the diet is far more complicated than originally believed. In fact, fat with the exception of a small number of bad fats is good for health. Furthermore, fat actually helps dieters refrain from overeating, because it leaves you feeling satiated and full of energy.

The Mediterranean diet isn't really a diet, it's simply the traditional way of eating in the Mediterranean region. Living very close to the sea, fish has long been a staple food of people living in the coastal regions of Spain, Portugal, France, Italy, Greece, and other countries. It has been known for a long time that people in these countries don't suffer from chronic diseases at the same rates that westerners do. In particular, rates of heart disease are quite low in these countries. Researchers soon noted that the Mediterranean diet actually included a large amount of fat. However, it was mostly unsaturated fat and fish oils. While there are some similarities to the DASH diet, the Mediterranean diet only provides suggestions of what to consume and doesn't give specific portions. This is because it's not a diet that has been designed by doctors, it's just a traditional cuisine.

The "pyramid" of the Mediterranean diet also has fruits and vegetables at the base, topped by whole grains like the DASH diet. However, there is no specification on how many servings to consume, basically, you eat until you're full. Meat can be consumed daily along with beans and legumes. Fish is consumed quite liberally at least twice per week, but often more than that. Avocados, which are consumed in strict moderation on the DASH diet because of its high-fat content, are eaten liberally on the Mediterranean diet. In addition, nuts can also be consumed liberally on the Mediterranean diet, and oils are consumed in abundance, but that would be specifically olive oil.

Why do this? Why not just stick to the Mediterranean diet? The reason is that high blood pressure is an independent risk factor for heart disease and stroke. That is, you can have low cholesterol, low triglycerides, high HDL, be thin and exercise, but if you have high blood pressure, you're still at elevated risk for having a heart attack or stroke. Controlling high blood pressure is one of the most important things you can do for your health.

Adding fat to the diet will help control diabetes, which may be the scourge of our time when it comes to public health concerns. The DASH diet really isn't suitable for dealing with diabetes, because low-fat diets are not really the best approach to use. Most people with pre-diabetes or diagnosed type-2 diabetes will find that even eating whole grains, or fruit, they will get blood sugar spikes. They will also probably find that following a low-fat diet like DASH, while it may help them control their weight and blood pressure, it won't do much to control their blood sugar. Here the Mediterranean diet steps in, with the high-fat content those with a tendency toward developing diabetes will find themselves having much better results. Those who are pre-diabetic may be able to avoid becoming full-blown type 2 diabetics. If you are already diagnosed with diabetes, without offering false hope, it is possible that following a strict version of the diet as outlined in this book may help you reduce or even get off your medications. This is something that you should discuss with your doctor.

The diet may also have dramatic effects on blood pressure. This can't be predicted ahead of time; some people are going to be more sensitive to salt than others. If you have high blood pressure and the diet isn't helping lower it, then adapt the low-sodium version of the DASH diet, which limits total sodium intake to 1,500 mg per day. If you are on blood pressure medication, this is something that you will need to discuss with your doctor before doing.

The DASH diet and the Mediterranean diet are both designed for long-term health. They can be considered more of a lifestyle than a diet. Don't be afraid to make adjustments to your eating plans as necessary to attain optimum health. We wish you the best of luck on your journey toward health and weight loss.